Manipulation

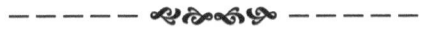

How to Secretly Persuade, Emotionally Influence and Manipulate Anyone Including Spotting Mind Control Tricks

David T Abbots

Copyright 2018 by David T Abbots - All rights reserved.

The follow book is reproduced below with the goal of providing information that is as accurate and reliable as possible. Regardless, purchasing this eBook can be seen as consent to the fact that both the publisher and the author of this book are in no way experts on the topics discussed within and that any recommendations or suggestions that are made herein are for entertainment purposes only. Professionals should be consulted as needed prior to undertaking any of the action endorsed herein.

This declaration is deemed fair and valid by both the American Bar Association and the Committee of Publishers Association and is legally binding throughout the United States.

Furthermore, the transmission, duplication or reproduction of any of the following work including specific information will be considered an illegal act irrespective of if it is done electronically or in print. This extends to creating a secondary or tertiary copy of the work or a recorded copy and is only allowed with express written consent from the Publisher. All additional right reserved.

The information in the following pages is broadly considered to be a truthful and accurate account of facts and as such any inattention, use or misuse of the information in question by the reader will render any resulting actions solely under their purview. There are no scenarios in which the publisher or the original author of this work can be in any fashion deemed liable for any hardship or damages that may befall them after undertaking information described herein.

Additionally, the information in the following pages is intended only for informational purposes and should thus be thought of as universal. As befitting its nature, it is presented without assurance regarding its prolonged validity or interim quality. Trademarks that are mentioned are done without written consent and can in no way be considered an endorsement from the trademark holder.

Your Free Gift

As a way of saying thank you for your purchase, I wanted to offer you a free bonus E-book called **5 Incredible Hypnotic Words To Influence Anyone**

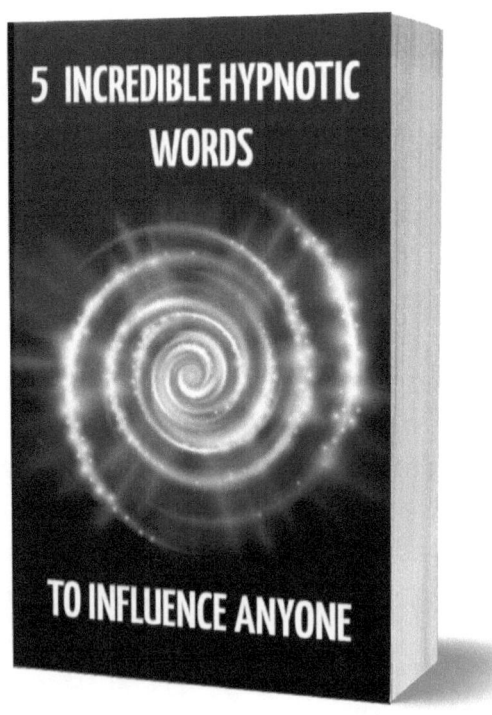

Download the free guide here: https://www.subscribepage.com/b1b5i8

If your trying to persuade or influence other people then words are the most important tool you have to master.

As Humans we interact with words, we shape the way we think through words, we express ourselves through words. Words evoke feelings and have the ability to talk to the lister's subconscious.

In this free guide, you'll discover 5 insanely effective words that you can easily use to start hypnotizing anyone in conversation.

Listen to this book for free

Do you want to be able to listen to this book whenever you want? Maybe whilst driving to work or running errands. It can be difficult nowadays to sit down and listen to a book. So I am really excited to let you know that this book is available in audio format. What's great is you can get this book for FREE as part of a 30-day audible trial. Thereafter if you don't want to stay an Audible member you can cancel, but keep the book.

Benefits of signing up to audible:
- After the trial, you get 1 free audiobook and 2 free audio originals each month
- Can roll over any unused credits
- Choose from over 425,000 + titles
- Listen anywhere with the Audible app and across multiple devices
- Keep your audiobooks forever, even if you cancel your membership

Click below to get started
Audible US - https://tinyurl.com/y55tluoj
Audible UK - https://tinyurl.com/y4n3y5s5
Audible FR - https://tinyurl.com/y4lyrkws
Audible DE - https://tinyurl.com/y34n5ejy

Table of Contents

Introduction 1

Chapter One: Manipulation and Mind Control Techniques 11

Chapter Two: Emotional Manipulation Techniques.. 35

Chapter Three: The Body Language of Manipulation 53

Chapter Four: Reading Body Language and Analyzing People 67

Chapter Five: Secret Social and Subconscious Manipulation Strategies 85

Conclusion 91

Introduction

Manipulation is primarily the art of getting people to do precisely what you want them to do without focusing on their needs and desires, and in extreme cases, even causing them harm. However, though manipulation has majorly negative undertones, it can be used for persuading and influencing people. It can consist of a series of techniques like charisma, trickery, misinformation, hypnotism, and wordplay.

The prime objective of manipulation is to trick people into doing what you want them to do without them realizing that they are being manipulated or being led into doing something. Sometimes, manipulation can be used to accomplish a positive outcome by turning the game when nothing else seems to be working.

For example, let's say you are due for a promotion and pay hike after working hard for your organization, but the firm just won't relent. When logical and other straight techniques don't

Manipulation

work, you may have to resort to manipulation to get your stingy employers to give you your due. In such situations, manipulation is used constructively to accomplish a positive goal when you can't break through another person's unreasonableness or stubbornness.

Knowingly or unknowingly, we've been practicing manipulation even before we started speaking. Babies want to be fed, kept clean, and put to sleep. Toddlers cry for toys until the parents give in. As an adolescent, we manipulate people to go on dates with us.

Manipulation originates from the primary belief that your requirements or desires come before everyone else's. For the manipulator, the world revolves around their needs and desires. However, manipulation can be lent a more positive angle when it is used to align you and other people's needs.

Unlike persuasion or influence, manipulation happens at a more subconscious level. It is done to change an individual's primary beliefs, feelings, and experiences for getting them to do what you want. It can be accomplished by using a range of techniques from verbal and non-

Introduction

verbal communication to hypnotism to smooth seduction techniques. Manipulation is essentially distorting an individual's perception of reality. The manipulator gets people to think in the direction he/she wants to.

If you've read Shakespeare's tragedies such as Othello or Macbeth, manipulation forms the central theme of their plot. The ingenious playwright understood manipulation in relationships, politics, and leadership even before there was a popular term for it.

In Othello, the villain Iago employs a bunch of vicious psychological tricks, including deception and craftily planned scenarios to get Othello to suspect his trusted chief

lieutenant Cassio so Iago can replace him. Lago creates a complex plot that leads Othello to believe that his ladylove Desdemona is cheating on him with the lieutenant. The villain uses his knowledge of psychology to climb his way into power by manipulating people's thoughts and circumstances to suit his quest for power.

Macbeth is another popular Shakespearean tragedy that is based on the theme of

Manipulation

manipulation. Lady Macbeth manipulates her husband using several psychological techniques to eliminate King Duncan and proclaim himself the ruler of the mighty Scottish throne. Macbeth then goes on a murderous rampage to protect himself from suspicion and enmity, which presents him a tyrant. The bloodbath ultimately led to the downfall and end of Macbeth and Lady Macbeth.

Lady Macbeth and the witch sisters use a series of manipulation strategies throughout the classic to instigate and encourage Macbeth into performing inhuman acts that eventually led to his doom. They manipulated Macbeth into thinking that he alone is capable of ruling the land, thus planting seeds of ambition, power, and hatred, which caused his and Lady Macbeth's end.

Is it possible to manipulate constructively or positively?

Yes, manipulation can be used positively and negatively depending on the end result—think about manipulating a perennially depressed person into seeing a counselor after failing to persuade him/her through other means. Then,

Introduction

imagine manipulating a drug addict or alcoholic into giving up the substance or alcohol. That isn't too bad, is it? You are using supposedly negative techniques to accomplish a positive goal.

Positive manipulation or persuasion/influence has been going on for ages. Religious leaders, political bigwigs, and social reformers attracted people like magnets through manipulation with their positive energy, ideas of humanity, equality, and brotherhood. That wouldn't qualify as tricky manipulation. They influenced people with their positive ideas, personalities, and examples to learn important life lessons.

There are multiple times in your life when you've wanted to transform someone's life for good. Yet, people may turn down your straight attempts to reach out to them owing to many reasons. In such cases, persuading or influencing people through the use of trickery or manipulation to fulfill a positive end for their own benefit may not be so bad. Irrespective of the techniques you use, your tactics cannot be termed devious or crafty.

Sometimes desperate times do indeed call for desperate measures. Using straightforward

Manipulation

approaches may not work all the time. The only way you can get someone to do something is by using backhand techniques. Your objective isn't to get the person to do what you want to fulfill a personal agenda. It is to move past a person's stubbornness and obstinacy.

Let us consider an example to see how manipulation can be used positively. You have a childhood buddy Ray whose wife has just left him for another man. Predictably, it has turned his life on its head. The two of you have been thick since childhood before Ray moved to another city for work. You get to know through a mutual friend that Ray has gone into severe depression, which has affected not just his personal life but also his work. His performance at work is abysmally down, and he could lose his job soon. Since you are old friends and concerned about Ray, you are worried about his depression and the subsequent effect it is having on his work.

You are aware that he is a primarily emotional, sensitive and psychologically weak person who wouldn't have taken this development very kindly. Like any good old childhood friend, you go over to meet Ray and talk to him about it. He

Introduction

shares his story with you, and you suggest he see a counselor.

Ray is adamant that he won't visit a counselor because he doesn't see how it can help bring back his wife, whom he loved dearly. You try to reason with him and tell him that it is not about getting his wife back. Rather, it is about getting a grip on his life and moving on. Again, he refuses to budge. He just doesn't understand how visiting a therapist or counselor can resolve his problem. His life is going more and more downhill with every passing day, and you just can't see him in letting his life slip away from his hands in this manner. You try to coerce, persuade, and convince him using every trick in the book, but he doesn't buy it!

How do you overcome this obstinacy and unreasonableness?

In absolute desperation, you tell him how your co-worker's wife left him, and he went into severe depression. You go on to list details about how the unfortunate event affected his performance at work. As a manipulator, you pick the right words, gestures, expressions, voice, theatrics, and emotions to let your friend know

Manipulation

that the co-worker really had a tough time coping with his depression. You launch into overdrive describing how it consumed his personal and professional life.

This is the point where you slowly introduce the idea of how your co-worker decided enough is enough and that he was going to take control of his life by seeking professional help. You booked an appointment for the co-worker with a counselor, and on your recommendation/suggestion, the co-worker agreed to see the counselor.

With the practiced tact of a manipulator, you inform Ray about how the co-worker's strong will and multiple beneficial counseling sessions helped him slowly to get his life back on track. You inform him going for regular therapy, and counseling sessions gave your co-worker the hope and courage to tackle the seemingly adverse situation in his life. What you are doing is stirring the right emotions within the person to get him to act in his best interests while moving past his unreasonableness and stubbornness.

Introduction

You are hoping that after hearing your co-worker's story, Ray is also moved into taking action. After listening to the story, Ray decides to see a counselor and starts going for regular therapy sessions. Slowly yet surely, you can see his life getting back on track. Ray appears more in control of his life, and his performance at work starts improving.

Here's the catch, my friends. None of what you told Ray is true. It is a cleverly spun tale and fabricated instance involving an imaginary co-worker. It involves lies, misinformation, and deception. However, is making up a story or manipulation in such a scenario so bad? You made it all up to push Ray into taking action. You manipulated your friend Ray into meeting a counselor and helped him move on. The aim is to enhance his psychological condition through trickery, manipulation, and lies. Sometimes, manipulation opens a small window through which an individual moves past his stubbornness to take action in the right direction.

Even when you are training an animal to "sit," "fetch," "jump," etc., by dangling their favorite treat, you are actually manipulating them to do what you want them to. Yes, it may be referred to

Manipulation

as training, but that's just a clever play of semantics. You may be training your dog to stay out of harm or lead a more disciplined life, which may be positive manipulation.

If you are a parent or have ever observed one, you know it is a herculean task to get kids to do something against their will. Parents are perpetually offering made up stories about angels, fairies, Santa Claus, monsters, and more to get them to do things that are good for them (the kids). Well, eating spinach doesn't give you superpowers, but sometimes that's the only way to get a stubborn toddler to eat it.

Subtle manipulation can be used for motivating and inspiring people for doing things that are good for them. Utilizing these approaches, you can transform someone's self-image, addiction, bad habits and more.

Think of manipulation as a work tool like a hammer. It can be used to hit a nail on the wall, or it can be used to destroy the wall. It is like holding a matchstick in your hand. You can light a candle for light, or you can start destruction by causing a fire.

Chapter One: Manipulation and Mind Control Techniques

Before we begin discussing ways to manipulate people by using mind control techniques, bear in mind that, on the whole, manipulation isn't considered a good way to accomplish a goal. Instead of using this mental trickery to fulfill evil personal agenda, use it for a positive purpose or to detect manipulation in your daily interactions. Protect yourself from manipulative folks and get people to accomplish more positive goals by applying these powerful persuasion/manipulation techniques.

World renowned social psychologist Robert B. Cialdini has mentioned six primary principles to change people's thoughts, feelings, and actions that, when practiced, help you become a powerful influencer and persuader.

Manipulation

1. Reciprocity

People have an innate need to return another person's favor. When someone buys you an expensive gift, you feel obliged to return an equally expensive gift or a valuable favor. If you want to get a person to do something, bring about a feeling of obligation in them. Keep reinforcing everything that you've been doing for a person over a period of time. Say something like, "Oh! Wouldn't you do the same for me or help me when needed?" in place of "Oh! It is nothing; please don't embarrass me by mentioning it." You are subtly planting the idea that in the future, you expect them to reciprocate by doing what you want.

2. Scarcity

When something is scarce, we tend to value it even more. This is a popular manipulation technique used by advertisers, marketers, and brand managers to get consumers to buy their products. Think "limited edition," "while stocks last," "limited period offer," "selected customers only," and more. When you position something as scarce, rare, or available for only a limited period, people tend to act with a greater sense of urgency and take immediate action.

3. Commitment and Consistency

Get people to do what you want them to do by getting them to commit. It is simpler to persuade them into doing what you want. For example, if you get someone to give something in writing or make a public declaration about their intention to do something, they can be held responsible or accountable for failing to do it. This increases your chances of getting them to do what you want them to do. People don't like going back on their words or being seen as someone who doesn't live up to their commitments.

4. Authority

Ever wondered why a majority of health, hygiene, and safety product promotions and advertisements have "authorities" or "experts" in a field waxing eloquent about how buyers will benefit from buying these products? Social media influencers get paid handsomely to promote products and services in the form of reviews or recommendations. People dig authority and expertise. If they view someone as an authoritative expert in a field, they are likelier to do what he/she tells them to do. If you want people to take a specific action, bring on board someone who they view as an authority. Get the expert to tell them what you want them to do. It works! Again, whether these methods are utilized to fulfill a negative or positive outcome is up to the person using them.

5. Liking

Answer this honestly. A very attractive, confident and friendly salesperson in a store is selling the same thing that another plain and slightly hesitant salesperson is selling in another store. Who will you purchase from? Though both are nice people, you will buy it from the person you like, and—correct me if I am wrong—a majority of people will like a person who comes across as attractive, charismatic, and friendly. Spend more time with a person to increase familiarity. Instead of asking your crush straight out for a date, get them to like you by hanging out as pals. There are fewer chances of a person refusing because you are now familiar with them, and they like you.

Chapter One: Manipulation and Mind Control Techniques

6. Social Proof

Whether you see this as a bane or a boon, people are wired to do what everyone else is doing. The herd mentality is deeply ingrained in the human mind since our hunting/gathering era. People invariably assume that because everyone is doing something, it must be the right thing to do. How many times have you been invited to a social gathering only to inquire who will be in attendance? There are higher chances of you attending when you realize everyone from your circle of friends, co-workers, or competitors are going to be there. There is a deep-seated fear of being left out. Why do companies and businesses ask for reviews from existing customers to attract new customers? Social validation!

18 Powerful Strategies for Manipulating People

We practice manipulation in some form or another throughout our lives, though its magnitude varies vastly. There are plenty of sneaky techniques, strategies and tricks to control people's minds and get them to do what you want.

Manipulation

How can you control another person's mind by bringing about a shift in their subconscious mind? Here are some powerful tips to control other people's thoughts, feelings, and actions without making them realize that they are being manipulated.

1. Establish Similarity

People instantly take to people who they perceive to be similar to them. It dates back to the primitive times when humans communicated their similarity with each other or being one among the same group through non-verbal communication. Establishing similarity works effectively until today. When you are trying to get people to do what you want or impress them, focus on creating familiarity.

People will develop a powerful sense of affiliation if you demonstrate that you are one among them through your voice, choice of words, and body language. This will increase your chances of getting them to do what you desire.

If you are trying to win over someone you've just met (a potential client or date), mirror their actions. Carefully notice the way they walk, talk,

Chapter One: Manipulation and Mind Control Techniques

hold their glass, lean against the bar and more to follow suit. Try using the same words and expressions they use. Observe the way they hold their glass. Sip on your drink a few seconds after they sip on theirs. If they shift their weight from one foot to another or lean against the wall in a specific manner, follow suit. Mirror their intonation, words, expressions, gestures, and posture.

Make the mirroring subtle and inconspicuous. The act shouldn't be too noticeable, or it may backfire, and the other person may think you are making fun of them. Mimicking can be offensive to the other person, and it'll only end up hurting your cause. This works especially well in a professional scenario where emotions rarely work.

2. Develop Charm and Charisma

Charisma is hard to explain but can be instantly identified in people when seen. Charm and charisma can help you impress people in a smooth/effortless manner to do what you want them to. They can seamlessly work their way into hypnotizing people with their charisma to think, speak, and act in a specific manner.

Manipulation

Practice developing a warm, inviting and congenial vibe. Stay approachable, friendly, and humorous (especially self-deprecating humor that makes you come across as more confident). Keep your body language open and flexible (more on manipulating people through body language later). Work on your conversation skills, appearance, and oratory skills to win people over. You should grab people's attention and arrest their interest through slick conversation skills. Learn the art of making small talk to establish a killer rapport with people.

People who are experts in manipulation almost always have excellent conversational skills. They will compliment people lavishly to win them over or make them feel exclusive/special. They'll look people in the eyes while talking with the intention of influencing people. If you want to manipulate a person into doing what you want, make them feel special. Give them the feeling that you are truly interested in their feelings, desires, and emotions. Demonstrate that you are going out of your way to understand them and care for their interests even if you don't actually care.

Chapter One: Manipulation and Mind Control Techniques

Confidence is another big attribute of charisma. Seasoned manipulators often have magnetic personalities and know the effect they wield over people. Confidence makes people more attractive. It reveals to the other person that you know what you are saying, which makes you more persuasive and believable. If you have complete faith in your abilities, you will be likelier to succeed when it comes to influencing people to think/behave like you or in another specific manner.

When people notice your confidence, they place greater trust and faith in you. They will take your actions seriously when they realize you know precisely what you are saying or doing. This comes only by practicing confidence. Be smooth talking and glib when you want to get people to do what you want, irrespective of whether you are speaking the truth.

3. Take Drama or Theater Lessons

One of the greater challenges when it comes to manipulating people is to master the right emotions, expressions, intonation, voice, words, and body language when you may not be feeling it. You are contriving or faking a specific set of actions to get the desired result.

You may have to pretend being distressed, unhappy, or disillusioned when you don't have your way to persuade people into giving in to your demands. Taking drama or theatre lessons is a clever way to sharpen your manipulation skills.

Master manipulators know how to master their emotions. Practice controlling your emotions and actions while trying to get people to do what you want. You may have to cry or appear elated in seconds. You'll have to learn to put up various acts according to the situational demands. Mastering the art of using your emotions, expressions, and actions at will is a valuable skill for any manipulator. Note: don't let people you are intending to manipulate know that you are taking acting lessons or your acts won't have much credibility or authenticity.

4. Practice Reading and Analyzing People

Every person has a unique personality, which means the same manipulation techniques may not work for everyone. You'll have to use distinct

Chapter One: Manipulation and Mind Control Techniques

emotional, psychological, and logical techniques to get people to respond in a specific manner based on their personalities.

Identify people's hot buttons or trigger points before attempting to manipulate them (much like the way salespersons do). What is their fundamental personality? How do they think, act, feel, and behave? What are their inherent desires, fears, and motivators? Take time to analyze people's personality before manipulating them. What moves them or makes them tick? Which is the best approach to get them to do what you want?

Identify people who are receptive to emotional responses, who are easier manipulation targets. Psychologically it is easy to manipulate people who display more emotional responses such as sympathy for other people, empathizing with other's problems, feeling disturbed when others are hurt, crying while watching sad movies, feeling a sense of compassion for animals and more. To get these people to do what you want, you have to awaken their emotions psychologically.

Manipulation

Similarly, other people are more prone to logical responses and therefore will respond more favorably to facts, figures, statistics, and other hard data. When you observe that a person keeps up with news reports, facts, and figures before making important decisions, use a more rational, persuasive, and composed approach. A calm and logical approach can work effectively when it comes to influencing people. Use a more calm, subtle, and logical approach that doesn't involve excessive use of emotions.

5. Fear-Relief Technique

This is a highly proven manipulation tactic that you've probably used knowingly or unknowingly at some juncture. Follow up an unreasonable request with a more realistic request to increase your chances of getting the other person to agree with you. This works at a deeply psychological level where the person places both the requests against each other and feels slightly relieved by the second request after being disturbed by the initial unreasonable one.

The feelings of confusion and tension are thwarted by the second request, thus increasing

Chapter One: Manipulation and Mind Control Techniques

your chances of getting someone to agree to your actual request.

Let us say for instance you want to seek permission from your boss to leave work early for the next couple of days. You ask your manager for permission to leave early for the next few months. When he/she appears taken aback by the idea, you immediately claim the opportunity to say something like, "Hey, Peter, no stress. Would you please allow me to leave early for the next couple of days?"

He/she will be relieved because this seems like a more reasonable request compared to the first one. The person will be more receptive to your request. Also, once he/she has refused something, it is more challenging to follow it up with another negative answer. The person will most likely relent to your request.

Fear-and-relief is a wicked psychological manipulative technique which works like a charm. It is considered essentially evil because it involves preying on an individual's emotions by causing him/her a great deal of anxiety and then abruptly relieving that built-up stress. The person becomes disarmed after the rise and drop

Manipulation

in emotions, which makes him/her less prone to make logical decisions. Thus, they are more likely to respond more positively to your request.

Here's a study that demonstrated how fear-relief works wonders when it comes to manipulating people.

These experiments listed in The Science of Social Influence and Will demonstrate how fear-relief manipulation works on a subtle level to accomplish the desired results. In one of the experiments, mall visitors were alarmed by a stranger who suddenly tapped them on their shoulder from behind. When people turned around, they found a blind man who wanted to know the time. After the fear and relief, the blind man's associates ask their targets to purchase and sign postcards for charitable causes. The rollercoaster of emotions got the targets to do things more effectively than control group participants who didn't go through the fear-relief manipulation.

The classic technique is evident in the bad-cop, good-cop routine. An authority scares the wits out of you, and another comes over and rescues you. Thus you become more open to sharing

Chapter One: Manipulation and Mind Control Techniques

information. Insurance salespersons use the technique all the time, and so do crafty managers. They will scare the shit out of you by informing you that your job is in jeopardy. Then, they'll request you to put in additional hours of overtime if you want to save your job.

6. Get Your Foot in the Door

The foot-in-the-door strategy was used by door-to-door salespersons in olden times when they tried to put their foot in the door to prevent people from banging the door on their faces. Today, the technique is used for establishing a rapport with people or breaking the ice by making a small request that is easy for them to fulfill. Later, you move in with the bigger and actual request very subtly. What you are doing is launching a series of positive replies.

This technique is the opposite of the earlier manipulation strategy. It is based on the psychological principle that once a person replies in the affirmative to your tiny and reasonable request, it will be tough for them to reply in the negative for what you actually want them to do.

7. Use Home Turf Advantage

When you are planning to get someone to do exactly what you want them to, arrange to meet on home ground to gain a clear psychological authority or advantage over them. When a physical space belongs to you, you subconsciously wield more control or authority in the situation.

It can be any place where you exercise greater psychological dominance (home, workplace, vehicle, etc.) to any other place where you feel a sense of familiarity, belongingness, and ownership. The other person should experience a sense of being on unfamiliar ground so they can rely on your confidence to make their decision.

This is exactly why friends and acquaintances who plan to sign you up for network marketing businesses will also ask you to join them for a presentation at their place or territory that is familiar to them over a space that belongs to you. They rely on the home ground advantage to get you to agree to their schemes and proposals.

Also, if you are negotiating a big business deal or getting a prospective client to agree to purchase

Chapter One: Manipulation and Mind Control Techniques

your products or services, it may work to your advantage if you get them to agree to come over to your workplace or a restaurant that is familiar to you (or where everyone from the server to the owners knows you well). What you are doing is giving yourself a psychological edge by negotiating on familiar ground.

8. Bribe

The powerful strategy of rewarding a person with the intention of getting them to return the favor can work well across situations. Reward a person psychologically, emotionally, or materially with something, so they feel compelled to return the obligation. When they do return the obligation, make sure it is by doing what you want them to.

Start by recognizing what your boss or partner wants, and do it for them. Don't forget to make it clear to them that you are doing them a favor, and when the time comes, you expect it to be returned. When you want them to do something for you, strike and remind them that it is time to give back.

While using this mind control or manipulation strategy, don't let it come across as emotional

Manipulation

blackmail or it'll backfire. The idea is not to let the other person know that you are manipulating them into acting in a particular way. Let it come across as you are genuinely trying to help the other person by going out of your way. This technique works well because the other person perceives a clear benefit initially and hence feels persuaded to give in.

For example, if you plan to ask your manager for a few days off work, prepare in advance to put in a few extra hours before asking him/her, especially if it's a busy time and he/she is likely to refuse your leave application. Stay up late and ensure he/she knows that you are going beyond your call of duty to fulfill the need of the hour. Subtly follow it up with your request of taking off from work for a few days. It is almost impossible for someone to refuse!

9. Use the setting to your advantage

Use the environment to your advantage by asking a person to do something for you at a place where they won't expect you to ask for it. Thus, you catch them off guard and disarm them before getting them to agree to your request. Don't be too caught up with "there is a place and

Chapter One: Manipulation and Mind Control Techniques

time for everything." Make the setting work in your favor by coming up with an unusual request.

For example, let's say you are out at the bar with your co-workers after work. Instead of asking for a favor in the office, use the chilled out and leisurely setting of the bar (when people are likelier to be in a more relaxed state) to get the person to agree to your request. When people are in a good mood or relaxed state of mind, they are less likely to refuse your requests. Go for the kill in a setting that is different from the expected setting to boost your chances of getting a positive response from the other person.

10. Gaslighting

Gaslighting has been extensively used in movies and books as a popular manipulation technique. It is a covert manipulation technique where a manipulator twists reality to meet their agenda. It is comprised of misleading the other person to believe (irrespective of whether it is their fault) that it is indeed their fault that they aren't able to perceive reality correctly.

The notion that they aren't able to see things correctly becomes so deeply embedded in their mind that they begin to question their perceptions and instead accept the manipulator's version of reality or truth. The technique is one of the most dangerous forms of manipulation because it is about making the other person feel so mentally incompetent that they stop having faith in themselves. It goes to the extent where they become mistrustful of people who oppose their perceptions because the ideas are so deeply sown in their psyche.

11. Rationalization

Rationalization is another effective technique through which a manipulator cleverly justifies their downright hurtful or inappropriate action. The technique works well because the justification offered is logical enough for a person to subscribe to it.

Rationalization accomplishes three primary purposes including removing resistance that manipulators may have about their not-so-appropriate acts, preventing other people from pointing fingers at them and assisting the

Chapter One: Manipulation and Mind Control Techniques

manipulator in justifying their actions in the eyes of the victim.

Manipulators who utilize the power of rationalization generally behave in a very affectionate manner. Suddenly, they'll become cold, hard, and distant. The victim is soon exhausted by their behavior, and when he or she confronts them or avoids them, they will start crying or screaming and launch into overdrive about how stressed, upset, and depressed they have been lately. The manipulator makes the other person feel miserable about confronting them when they are clearly not in the right frame of mind.

The other person, not you, becomes the bad person when someone confronts you for your inappropriate behavior. The victim becomes the insensitive person instead of you. Manipulators move people to tears with how stressful and tough their life really is. They are adept at playing the victim and even justifying their terrible actions by blaming it on other people through rationalization rather than accepting the blame for their actions.

12. Master Your Own Emotions Before Preying on Other People's Feelings

This is last but certainly not the least. To be a class act manipulator, you have to have complete control over your feelings and emotions. You have to make people like you by coming across as positive and friendly all the time. As a manipulator or persuader, you will be required to get people to think, feel and act in a certain way. This requires you to be completely in control of your emotions.

You cannot be swayed by your emotions if you are aiming to control someone else's feelings. If you don't learn to master your emotions, you may end up being manipulated instead of manipulating others. Avoid falling into the plan you create for others and aim to create fear, uncertainty, or sympathy in others while being completely in control of your own feelings and emotions.

Manipulation is all about controlling and directing other people's feelings and emotions in a specific manner. Manipulators are compelled to exercise control over a situation to covertly or openly control other people's thoughts, feelings,

Chapter One: Manipulation and Mind Control Techniques

and actions. For example, you will make someone believe that they are overreacting to a situation when they are clearly not. Controlling other people's actions, feelings, and thoughts becomes easier when you are control of your own thought patterns and emotions.

Chapter Two: Emotional Manipulation Techniques

I think we've all forgotten how many times we've been told if we love someone we'll do things their way (read: go to a specific place to eat or go to the games over movies). Yes, that is the potency of raw emotions. It can be used constructively and destructively to get people to do what we want them to. Emotional manipulation happens when you leverage other people's feelings and emotions to your advantage or to accomplish an overall good. Again, it's a double-edged sword that can be used to fulfill some positive and negative intentions.

Here are some powerful emotional manipulation techniques:

Playing on People's Fears

Emotional manipulators tend to exaggerate facts or selectively highlight facts/reality/statistics to induce a sense of fear in their victims. For instance, a person who doesn't want their partner to pursue a full-time career outside their home and raise children instead may say something along the lines that, "research reveals 70 percent of all relationships break up when both partners pursue full-time jobs."

There can be other reasons too, but the manipulator chooses to create fear or a sense of insecurity by highlighting a single aspect to get their partner to act in a specific manner. This helps them play on the other person's fears that if they indeed give in to their ambition, they may end up losing the relationship.

Make the Other Person Feel Guilty

A majority of emotional manipulation techniques involve stirring a sense of guilt within the other person. Practiced manipulators know how to make the other person feel guilty to fulfill their own agenda. For instance, if someone brings up a grievance that is bothering them for a while, emotional manipulators will make them feel guilty for even making an issue out of a non-issue.

Chapter Two: Emotional Manipulation Techniques

Again, if they don't speak, emotional manipulators will make them feel guilty about hiding their feelings or not having a frank, straightforward conversation. As a manipulator, you keep brewing guilt in the other person irrespective of their thoughts and actions. Anything the other person does is attributed to them, so they are overcome by a strong sense of guilt and finally give in to your demands. Building a sense of guilt is one of the most powerful ways to get a person to obey you.

This works even more effectively on people who are not very sure of themselves or possess low self-confidence/self-esteem or are essentially indecisive. For example, if you want to get a friend to do exactly what you want, list everything you've done to help them, followed immediately by a mention of the times they've completely let you down.

You can also stir up an overpowering feeling of guilt within your partner by saying things such as, "it is okay, one can't expect anything different from you." This makes them feel like they are letting you down all the time, and that you can't expect anything else from them.

Manipulation

Observe how some seniors induce a strong sense of guilt in their children by emphasizing the fact that they (the children) don't spend time with their parents despite knowing that they aren't going to live for long. The children may be busy with their own hectic schedules and make time whenever possible.

Similarly, if parents don't allow their teenagers to go on a camp or a night out with friends, the adolescents will make their parents feel guilty for being overprotective and not allowing them to negotiate the world on their own. We use emotional manipulation in several ways throughout our lives. Only the intention and intensity varies from person to person.

I am sure you know someone who plays victim all the time even if life isn't as hard as they imagine it to be. These people will use their helplessness to act like victims and make others feel guilty to get them to do what they (the guilt-trippers) want. They give others a feeling that their fate is often in other people's hands. The other person then feels responsible for them, which induces a deep sense of guilt. They feel terribly guilty about refusing this person because the manipulator has craftily presented

Chapter Two: Emotional Manipulation Techniques

themselves as someone who needs help, and who'll be completely lost if you don't help them. The other person will invariably feel bad and do exactly what you want them to because they start feeling responsible for your fate and sense of helplessness.

Challenge the Other Person's Sense of Reality

Emotional manipulation also involves challenging or belittling the person's understanding of reality. Manipulators are skilled liars and deceivers. They possess the ability to confidently tell someone that something happened even though it may not have happened and something didn't happen when it may have happened. They can change someone's perception of reality by playing around with facts in a sneaky manner.

The victim of their manipulation will begin questioning their own perception of reality or sanity. For instance, if someone suspects the manipulator of having an affair and questions them about it, the manipulator will not only deny it but also turn the game around by making the other person feel guilty about doubting them.

Manipulation

They'll make the other person come across as crazy, suspicious, insecure, and possessive, owing to which the person may start questioning their own sanity or sense of reality.

Play The Victim

Seasoned manipulators put on the victim's garb with ease. If you plan to manipulate people emotionally, one of the most powerful ways is to act like a victim or behave like it is never your fault. Irrespective of who is at fault, manipulators will always blame their actions or shortcomings on others.

Focus on how someone made you do something even though you didn't necessarily want to do it. If the manipulator is hurt, upset or angry, the other person is blamed for hurting them. In short, manipulators do not accept any accountability from their actions.

Let us consider an example; If a regular person forgets their anniversary and the partner gets upset, he/she will apologize profusely to the partner and attempt to make up for it by doing something special for the partner.

Chapter Two: Emotional Manipulation Techniques

However, a manipulator will not just fail to accept their mistake, they will, in turn, make the partner feel guilty about blaming them for such a trivial matter when they've been stressed at work and have tons of things to remember. I know of people who will go even beyond that and remind the partner about all the instances where they've forgotten important things as a justification for their blunder.

One-upmanship

One-upmanship games are common among manipulators. Irrespective of how big other people's challenges and problems are, as a manipulator, your challenges and problems should always be pitched as worse. The idea is to undermine the genuineness of another person's problems by constantly playing up your issues as greater than theirs.

You make other people feel guilty for complaining about non-existing issues when you are fighting bigger battles. The idea is to make the other person feel like they don't have a reason to complain, while it is your right to focus on your rather "serious" issues. You want the other person to stop complaining and stay one-up during every situation, even when it comes to playing the victim.

Know Their Emotional Hot Buttons

One of the best ways of emotionally manipulating people is to know their emotional triggers or hot buttons. Everyone has their weak spots that can be used to get them to do what we want. Manipulation is about identifying these weak spots and using them to your advantage to get the person to do what you want.

For instance, if you know that a person is unsure or slightly conscious about their appearance, play on their insecurity by passing remarks about their weight, clothes, or appearance. Again, if someone is not confident about their public speaking or presentation skills, play on this fear by informing them about how difficult and judgmental the listeners are. Use the awareness of other people's emotions to get them to do what you want by leveraging them smartly.

Induce an Inferiority Complex

Emotional manipulators engage in decreasing a person's sense of self-worth or undermine their

Chapter Two: Emotional Manipulation Techniques

belief in themselves by judging, analyzing or criticizing the person. The objective is to marginalize, ridicule or dismiss a person constantly in an attempt to gain a sort of psychological dominance over them.

The objective is to make the other person feel off-balance, inferior and inadequate to get them to act in the way you want. When other people stop believing in their abilities or sanity, you have more control over their thoughts, feelings, and actions.

Emotional manipulators will intentionally plant the feeling that something isn't quite right with the other person to shake their sanity or sense of self-belief to fulfill an agenda. They'll make the victim feel like nothing they ever do is going to be enough. Importantly, the emotional manipulator will concentrate on the victim's weaknesses without offering positive feedback or constructive solutions, and guide them to overcome their weakness in meaningful ways.

The Silent Treatment

Another powerful manipulation weapon is the silent treatment. Emotional manipulators have mastered the art of giving people the silent treatment to pressure people into doing what they want. They will purposefully make a person wait and plant seeds of doubt and uncertainty within the person's mind. Emotional manipulators utilize the power of silence to keep their victims emotionally unsure or deprived.

The silent treatment can be used as a tool to encourage people into doing what you want them to do. You refuse to acknowledge their existence or make them feel inadequate to accomplish your objectives. If the victim's actions do not match that of the manipulator, the manipulator can convey their disappointment by penalizing the victim with the silent treatment.

Use Humor to Disempower People

Emotional manipulators use the power of humor to pick on people's perceived limitations or weaknesses in an attempt to disempower them or make them feel inadequate. Have you ever noticed how sometimes people make critical or caustic remarks about their friends or family in the disguise of humor? The objective is to make the other person feel insecure or inadequate.

Chapter Two: Emotional Manipulation Techniques

Emotional manipulators aim to throw their victims off guard by playing on their limitations and weaknesses. The remarks may appear humorous on the face of it and can target anything from the individual's appearance to their abilities to their smartphone. They may make fun of anything from the fact that you walked in late to the clothes you are wearing—with a clear intention of throwing you off balance or making you feel miserable about yourself.

This is a way to gain a psychological edge over the other person by undermining their sense of self-worth. The person starts feeling inferior, which disempowers them on a subconscious level and makes them more open to control or dominance.

Flattery

This almost always works like a charm if you do it right. Flattering words and compliments have the potential to move anyone's heart, but the intentions behind those words may not always be noble. Flattery is a weapon of attack for several manipulators to persuade people into fulfilling their personal agenda. As a tool of manipulation, flattery is used magnificently well by salespersons. To make this even more effective, make your compliments specific.

For example, rather than saying "your presentation was really good today," say, "I loved the ease with which you handled objections" or "I loved your closing statements." Specific compliments hit the nail on the head. For example, let us say you are in an apparel store trying something that you think doesn't look too good on you. However, the salesperson walks in and says, "Wow blue is indeed your color, this looks fabulous on you." What is your reaction? Don't you feel influenced to buy it immediately? There is a quick shift in your thought process. Flattery is a sneaky little trick to sweep others off their feet and get them to do what you want.

Ignorance or Helplessness

Helplessness and ignorance is another powerful tool used by manipulators to persuade people into doing what they want. You'll feign or pretend that you are not able to do things and use helplessness as an emotional manipulation trick to win other people's sympathy.

Chapter Two: Emotional Manipulation Techniques

Sometimes, use the excuse "you're better than me" or "smarter than me" to get someone to do something for you. However, ensure that you don't use this tactic frequently or people will see through your game.

Create a Sense of Urgency and Alarm

"Sale ends today" or "if you can't make a decision today, I am not staying here anymore" are typical phrases used by manipulators to get people to act by creating a sense of urgency. They may create a fake sense of panic or urgency to push people into taking action. When people feel like they don't have much time or they'll miss out on something important if they don't take action, their chances of doing something increases.

Use People's Commitments and Promises against Them

Who doesn't fancy being a "man of their word" by sticking to what they say? However, manipulators will cleverly use this trick to get people to do what they want by using their words against them. Life keeps changing, and people's promises keep fluctuating. However, if you are a smart manipulator, you will know how to use people's commitments and words to get them to do what you want. Even though things may have changed and it isn't possible to do what people earlier stated, use their words as an emotional manipulation tactic to get them to do what you want. Bring up their promise several times to let people know that they've got to do what they promised or they run the risk of being seen as someone who doesn't live up to their word or commitment.

Overcome trust issues

If someone has been manipulated several times before, they will most likely not trust people again. If trust is a major issue, nix it by sharing something private and personal with your target. It is all the more effective if the secret is relevant to the person or if they perceive that you trust them enough to share something so personal with them. Whether the story is true or not is irrelevant. You are focusing on winning the person's trust by demonstrating your faith in them. Again, putting on act is the clinching factor.

Chapter Two: Emotional Manipulation Techniques

Sugarcoat negative manipulation as altruism

Approach everything in a friendly and positive manner. Negativity doesn't make you an efficient manipulator. The key is to come across as a wonderful person who cares about others. Negative actions such as blaming, criticizing and yelling at another person should always be sugarcoated with altruism. Painting yourself as an altruistic person saves you from acquiring the label of a manipulator. People seldom despise someone who claims to care for them and wants the best for them.

For example, let us say you feel the need to yell at the other person for not taking an action you asked them to take. If you frame this as something you wanted them to do, you'll run the risk of coming across as selfish, self-centered, manipulative, etc. However, if you present the same thing as a way of helping them, the other person will feel you are acting in their interest.

Let us say as a boss, you give your employee some additional work to complete back home during the weekend which you were supposed to complete during the week. The employee didn't

Manipulation

finish it, and if you felt the need to yell at him/her for not getting your work done, you will naturally come across as selfish or self-centered. However, if you present it as something that will affect the employee's appraisals, reviews, chances of promotions, etc., you come across as a hero who cares about the employee's professional success and wants him/her to perform well or impress the management. Thus you are sugarcoating your own selfish desires as altruism.

If you are prone to outbursts, you'll have to learn to get a good grip on your emotions. Manipulation and emotional outbursts do not go well together. It may help you in a few instances, but in the long run, positive manipulation is more effective than negative manipulation techniques. If you do give in to an outburst, apologize to the person by stating that you were overcome by emotions because you care about him/her or are acting in their best interests. Never fail to remind the target that you will always be there for them.

Chapter Two: Emotional Manipulation Techniques

Act normal when you are caught manipulating

Several newbie manipulators falter when it comes to responding when their manipulative acts are discovered. When someone calls out your manipulative actions, the most terrible thing to do is engage in a more manipulative behavior. Stay normal or composed when someone calls out to your behavior.

Allow the other person to control the situation while you stay passive. Avoid defending your actions. The sole way to wriggle out of the situation is to stir doubt and make this doubt work to your benefit in the minds of your victims. Appear genuinely shocked and revolted. Create a shocked expression and make the other person feel guilty about their assumption. In a majority of the cases, people will start questioning their own assumptions, especially if you are well-known to them. They will latch on to any reason to believe in your positive virtues.

Manipulation

Learn More About Psychology and Neuroscience

Know more about psychology, human behavior, and neuroscience to manipulate people more effectively. You should have a fundamental understanding of how people think and behave if you desire to be a powerful manipulator. Sure, all the tips mentioned here are going to make you an effective manipulator, but you need a deeper understanding of human psychology to know which manipulation principles to apply in which situation, and to manipulate people effortlessly.

Chapter Three:
The Body Language of Manipulation

Manipulation is about persuading people to do what you want them to, which involves plenty of people influencing skills. Non-verbal communication comprises expressions, gestures, posture, walk, leg movements, voice, tone, etc. and is responsible for a major part of the communication process.

According to research conducted by Dr. Albert Mehrabian, only 7 percent of our communication happens through words. About 55 percent of the entire communication happens through body language and 38 percent through our voice. Now you can imagine why people insist that you meet them in person (and not over the phone) when they want to share something important with you. Body language and voice makes up a huge chunk of the communication process, which means manipulators need to master these elements to convince or persuade people to do what they want.

The manner in which you convey certain concepts, thoughts, emotions, facts, and feelings is going to influence other people's decisions. Communication skills are important when it comes to influencing people to do what you desire or take the required action. Hone your manipulation skills by mastering powerful communication techniques to come across as more persuasive, inspiring and influential.

Here are some secret tips to use when making non-verbal communication skills, including body language and voice for manipulating people into doing what you want them to do.

1. Let the other person talk first to establish a baseline.

When you are attempting to get someone to take a specific action (for instance: purchase from you), allow them to talk first. This way you get a chance to set a baseline for their behavior and detect their weaknesses that you can play on later. The personality or behavior baseline will give you a clear idea about thoughts, actions,

Chapter Three: The Body Language of Manipulation

motivators, needs, feelings, and behavior to help you determine their strengths, weaknesses, and goals. I'd say, go one step ahead and create a questionnaire to get the answers you are looking for.

2. Listen to people.

Manipulators must not just be excellent speakers. They must also be exceptional listeners. Practice active listening to know exactly what a person wants. It'll also give you a clear idea of a person's personality, needs, and wants. Listening to a person arms you with the power to come up with an appropriate response to what they are saying. For example, a prospective buyer or client may not need to purchase from you currently or may be considering purchasing from a competitor, and by not listening to them you are missing out on important bits of information.

If you miss this important information, you will not be able to handle their objections effectively. Since you haven't heard about their reference to a competitor, you won't be able to do a comparative analysis later to establish how your product is superior over a competitor's.

Manipulation

To make yourself more likable and accessible to people, acknowledge what people are saying by nodding or saying "hmms" or imitating their expression. You can also paraphrase what the person said to ensure you've heard it right. "Mr. XYZ if I get you correctly, you are not considering buying this product right now because you want to do a comparison with our competitor's prices, products, and features too? Is that correct?" Resist the urge to interrupt the other person while speaking and don't jump to offer solutions before the person finishes talking.

Even if we don't realize or admit it, all of us drift off after a point of time. Ask questions and repeat the last few words to clarify important points or give the other person the idea that you are keenly listening to or interested in them. Listen to people with an open mind without judging what they are saying.

Avoid being a conversation hijacker. Sometimes, your thinking will be quicker than the other person's pace of speech. You'll be tempted to finish their sentence for them while they are still grappling for the right words. This again does not give the other person a chance to finish what they are saying, and you may miss important bits

Chapter Three: The Body Language of Manipulation

of information. Don't listen to respond or start constructing your responses while listening. Listen to understand.

This will give you a greater edge while manipulating people. Try to remember what people say with the help of keywords or create a mental visual to better remember what they spoke.

3. Body language

Keep your body language confident, authoritative, poised, and self-assured. People buy your body language before they buy your words when they meet you for the first time. They are likelier to be taken in by a confident body language and voice. If your body language or voice is filled with hesitation or self-doubt, there's a slim chance others will accept what you are asking them to do.

- Manipulators are adept at the art of looking people in the eyes while speaking to come across as genuine and honest. While talking to people, face them and maintain eye contact all through the conversation. Constantly shifting your gaze away from the person makes appear dishonest. Again, fixating your gaze on a person makes you come across as intimidating. The best part is to look away briefly from time to time.

- A smile works wonderfully when it comes to establishing a rapport or a feeling of belongingness or similarity on a subconscious level. Boost your likability factor by having a smile plastered on your face permanently.

- Always lean slightly towards the person you are talking to. This reveals attentiveness and interest on your part. The head should be tilted towards them or in their direction while maintaining a healthy distance between the face. Point your feet towards them rather than the exit or the opposite direction!

Avoid invading a person's private space by getting too close to them physically. You should leave a gap of at least four feet between you and the other person. Just tilt your body in their direction or lean over a tabletop to reveal your interest in

Chapter Three: The Body Language of Manipulation

them while communicating/interacting with them.

- Stay attentive, unruffled, and relaxed. Avoid tapping your feet or fidgeting with your hands. It conveys the message that you are nervous or disinterested in what they are saying. Keep your feet and hands in a more relaxed position without being too conscious of it. Nervousness and manipulation/persuasion never go together.

- One super way of enhancing body language is to practice in front of a mirror. It allows you to determine how you appear to other people and what changes can be made to make your communication and presentation skills even more impactful. Notice your expressions, gestures, walk, posture and more. Do they have the intended effect on people? Do you appear calm, confident, persuasive, and self-assured while speaking? Does your speech inspire people to take immediate action?

Manipulation

When you meet someone for the first time, set your subconscious authority by offering a firm, assertive, and power-packed handshake. A limp and lifeless handshake communicates nervousness, uncertainty, and lack of confidence. It is easy for the other person to gain a psychological dominance over you, which will make it tough for you to manipulate him or her. Similarly, a crushing handshake indicates aggressiveness or absolute dominance.

- Amy Cuddy, a renowned social psychologist has mentioned a list of how to use specific power poses to your advantage in a TED Talk. The power postures will not just boost your testosterone levels but also decrease the body's cortisol levels in less than two minutes. These poses are believed to have a considerable impact on our thoughts, feelings, and actions on a very subconscious level. They give the message of the power of authority to the other person.

Chapter Three: The Body Language of Manipulation

A majority of these postures involve occupying more physical space by broadening your frame to make yourself appear powerful and bigger. When you take up greater physical space, you subconsciously establish yourself as a larger or more authoritative/dominant person.

While standing, expand your stance by keeping the feet apart. You will appear less nervous and more in control of the situation. Holding your feet together will make you come across as nervous and unsure.

- Research in the field of brain imaging has revealed that our brain's Broca area is responsible for speech stimulation within the body. This happens not just when we are talking but also while performing gestures such as moving our hands. Thus, our speech and hand gestures are more intricately woven than we realize. Thus by engaging your hands through gestures, you can facilitate your thoughts, ideas, and words.

Manipulation

> Some of the world's best speakers move their hands in animated gestures to make an arresting impact on their listeners. Your speech, thoughts, presentation, and clarity will be significantly enhanced if you use gestures. Eventually, you'll come across as more persuasive and convincing.

- Establish a quick rapport with the other person if you want to influence him/her into doing what you want with the help of body language. Face them directly while talking and be attentive while speaking. This will align your body language with their verbal and non-verbal communication pattern, which is especially helpful while addressing a group. When you want to influence or manipulate people into doing something, it is important to align with their body language and show them you are completely attentive and attuned to them through verbal and non-verbal signals.

4. Voice

Manipulators or persuaders/influencers generally have a more relaxed voice with a low

Chapter Three: The Body Language of Manipulation

pitch and assertive tone. Always speak in a low and assertive tone to come across as more authoritative rather than talking in a squeaky, high-pitched voice. The voice shouldn't rise when the sentence ends. It reveals doubt or uncertainty. It comes across as if you are asking a question or raising a doubt about something rather than making an assertive or authoritative statement. Allow your voice to completely relax before making an important presentation.

Maintain an assertive arc that works wonderfully well when it comes to manipulating/persuading people. The voice starts on a gentle note, while the pitch rises in the middle of a sentence, and eventually cascades at the end of the sentence.

A person's voice tone reveals plenty about how a person is feeling. If you don't speak in a consistent or even tone, it comes across as if you are concealing emotions or are not in control of your emotions such as nervousness, anger, and disappointment. Know when to pause to create the intended impact. When you make a powerful statement, pause to allow the idea to sink in!

Also, emphasize the right words to create the desired effect. Emphasizing the right words lends more impact and greater clarity to your communication, which is important for getting someone to take the required action.

An animated voice along the lines of voiceover artists or radio personalities works well when it comes to lending more punch to your message. Don't speak in a flat monotone throughout a speech or conversation. Vary it by lowering or elevating the pitch for creating the desired histrionics. One tip is to listen to famous radio presenters to understand how they modulate or play with their voice to evoke the desired emotions among listeners.

Volume depends on the people you are addressing. While addressing a big audience, keep it loud and authoritative. However, if it's a one-on-one conversation, speak in a low and soft tone.

5. Appearance

An attractive and pleasant appearance adds to your likeability factor and charisma. We discussed earlier how you are likelier to purchase from a person who is more physically attractive than someone who is plain-looking. Basic

Chapter Three: The Body Language of Manipulation

hygiene is the essence of being presentable, likable, and charismatic. People who smell good attract others like magnets.

Humans are drawn to clean, well-groomed and hygienic people on a primordial level. At a fundamental level, it is easier to manipulate people if you smell good and are clean. It will be challenging to manipulate people if you stink or appear untidy or unclean. Being well-groomed and hygienic doesn't require much effort. Shower, groom your hair neatly and wear a nice smelling fragrance.

Have a neat and well-groomed haircut that suits your face. The presentation of your hair impacts your overall appearance. Your haircut or hairstyle is one of the initial things a person notices about you when you try to influence them. Dress well if you want to make a favorable impact on people and appear confident.

Wearing well-cut outfits with flattering fits will make you look good. And we all know when we look and feel good about ourselves, our confidence shoots up several fold. Looking good will make you come across as more confident, self-assured, and influential. People will be more

Manipulation

likely to look up to you and agree with what you say if you come across as confident and in control. Try taking someone whose appearance or attire you do not like seriously. It just won't click.

Chapter Four: Reading Body Language and Analyzing People

To manipulate people, you've got to dive right into their mind and understand what they are thinking. Master manipulators are adept at the art of speed reading people through verbal and non-verbal signals. Only when you understand people are you able to determine the right approach for manipulating them. For instance, some people are more prone to emotional responses and reactions and emotional manipulation may work well for them. Similarly, others may be more logical by nature. For such people, logical manipulation techniques may work more effectively.

You can determine your own body language, words, expressions, gestures, and more to manipulate people once you know how they are thinking or feeling. Here are some of the best body language tips to read people.

Crossed Arms And Legs

Folded legs and arms are a nonverbal signal of a subconscious barrier. It demonstrates that the other person is psychologically closed to what you are speaking or isn't interested or trustful of what you are saying. Sometimes, they may have a smile on their face, or they may speak in a friendly manner. However, their non-verbal gestures may reveal a different story about their psychological thought process.

Crossing arms and legs is a signal of creating a physical or psychological subconscious barrier between the speaker and listener. When you get a feeling that the person is shutting off from what you are saying by crossing their hands and legs, change the topic to something that is of interest to them. Allow the other person to get into a more relaxed frame of mind or open up a bit before getting back to the original topic. The process happens so subconsciously that the other person isn't even aware of it.

Real Smiles

How can you distinguish a genuine smile from a fake one? Here's the deal. Our mouths can often

Chapter Four: Reading Body Language and Analyzing People

contrive smiles even when we don't feel like smiling. However, the eyes and the region around the eyes cannot deceive since it's a very subconscious driven microexpression.

When a person is genuinely smiling, it is evident in their eyes. A real smile reaches the eye and causes the skin around the eyes to form wrinkles or crow's feet. People fake smiles to hide their true feelings. However, seasoned manipulators will look for crinkles near the eye region to determine if the person is indeed happy or simply faking delight.

Eyes Don't Lie

When people don't hold their gaze for too long or don't maintain steady eye contact, they may be lying to you. When people speak the truth, they confidently hold the other person's gaze. Remember when your parents or teachers told you to look into their eyes while speaking. However, the knowledge that people who do not look you in the eye has become so common and widely shared that liars and deceivers can now intentionally or purposefully hold their gaze for long.

Manipulation

When a person is holding their gaze continuously without looking away even occasionally, there may be something amiss. The ideal way is to maintain eye contact with a person while looking away at regular intervals.

Increased Nodding

If a person is nodding more than required or nodding in a highly exaggerated way, he or she is worried or concerned about your approval. This can be used to your advantage when it comes to manipulating the person. While addressing a group, always look out for people who are nodding excessively. They are the ones who are worried about your impression of them. These people are subconsciously seeking your approval, which makes them easy manipulation targets.

Stress

How does one detect internal stress through a person's body language? Some of the most common signs of stress are clenched jaws, furrowed brows, fidgeting fingers, and stiff necks. Irrespective of what someone is saying, they may be under some discomfort.

Chapter Four: Reading Body Language and Analyzing People

They may not be very comfortable discussing the topic or thinking about a problem that is clearly causing them anxiety. This is a quick opportunity to seize and play savior if you want to get them to do something.

Catch signs of stress in people to reach out to them and present yourself as a solution to their problems, and eventually persuade or manipulate them into doing what you want! The objective of reading people's body language is to observe a clear difference between their words and body language to understand how they are truly thinking or feeling.

Nervousness

Excessive blinking, fidgeting with their hands, tapping feet, and increased facial movements are all signs of nervousness. Closely observe how people develop jittery feet when they are nervous.

Feet Direction

Watch the direction of a person's feet while communicating with them. The direction of their feet can reveal a lot about what they are thinking at a subconscious level. Since the feet are the most ignored or overlooked part of the body, people do not focus too much on their foot movements or direction. This makes it a powerful subconscious thought-determining mechanism.

If a person's feet are pointed towards the door or exit, they are looking to run away from the place at the first given opportunity. However, if a person's feet are pointed in your direction, they are hooked to the conversation. Whenever you are engaged in an interesting conversation with a person, your foot will involuntarily move forward. It happens at such a subconscious level, which makes it near dependable.

Eye Movements

Our eye movements are closely connected with specific regions of the brain. When you move your eyes in a particular direction, it reveals the brain function that is active. For instance, if you are asked to recall a familiar childhood sound, your eyes will dart slightly up and towards the left to visualize a person or thing that emitted the sound. Then, they move slightly downwards

Chapter Four: Reading Body Language and Analyzing People

followed by movement to the right when you begin recalling the sound or voice.

Our eye movements have a clear pattern (much of NLP or Neuro Linguistic Programming is based on reading people through their eye movements) based on the brain function that is active at a particular time. The brain nerves are closely linked with our eyes to cause very split-second micro eye movements that when you closely observe tell a lot about a person's thought patterns. This is vital information for a manipulator.

When you ask someone something that they can't easily recollect, they eyes will dart to the upper-left direction. This simply indicates that they are attempting to pull out information from past memory. It is widely established that people who are visual learners rely on their visual memory for extracting information. Similarly, if an individual moves their eyes to the upper-left when they are confronted with something, they are not recalling information but rather making it up. In short, they are not telling the truth or answering from memory. Rather, they are trying to make stories.

Manipulation

If they move their eyes to the upper right direction when they are asked something, people are most likely speaking the truth because they are trying to recollect information from their memory before replying. Take for instance: you ask a person where they are returning from, and he/she looks to the upper left instead of upper right, he/she is not recollecting facts but constructing them. This is important information when it comes to manipulating people.

When a person is fighting an internal dilemma, he/she will most likely look towards their left collarbone. This indicates that an individual is thinking deeply about something or engaged in an internal dialogue. For instance, when you confront a person, he or she may be stuck in a dilemma between speaking the truth and lying.

Similarly, when a person darts their eyes quickly from one side to another, it is an indication of telling lies or seeking some form of escape from the situation. They may be afraid of being caught. The person is most likely creating conspiracies in his/her mind.

Chapter Four: Reading Body Language and Analyzing People

When people remember a specific physical sensation experience, their eyes move towards the lower right side. Try to imagine the physical sensation of satin on your skin while keeping your eyes shut. The eyes will reflexively move towards the lower right side.

Attraction

If a person is deeply attracted to you or fixated on a conversation with you, the size of their pupil will invariably expand. Their pupil's contract when the subject of the conversation is boring or the conversation doesn't excite them.

Also, people who are attracted to you may lean in your direction or have their feet pointed towards you. Blinking more than the average blinking rate is also seen as a sign of attraction. If a person blinks over 8-10 times a minute, there's a high chance they are attracted to you. These movements occur at a subconscious level while they are trying to internally process feelings of attraction, which is exactly why blinking is connected with flirting in popular culture.

When someone is charmed by you, their eyes will shine. There is an innately psychological reason behind this. When a person is attracted to someone, their eyes turn a little moist. This reflects more light. Thus, shining eyes along with other above-mentioned clues are an indication of attraction.

Avoiding Errors While Reading Body Language Correctly

Being a master manipulator is about reading people's body language accurately while avoiding potential errors. When you read people correctly, you can tailor your responses according to their thoughts, feelings, and emotions to persuade them into doing exactly what you want. Here are some tips for spotting potential fallacies while reading body language.

Establish a Baseline For Reading People

It is important for establishing a baseline for people's behavior to read them accurately. If you are meeting someone for the first time, you may not really have the opportunity to establish a baseline. However, as far as possible, knowing more about an individual's personality or behavior allows you to gain more reliable information about them through their body

Chapter Four: Reading Body Language and Analyzing People

language. You'll get a more in-depth, accurate, and comprehensive overview of their personality.

For example, let us say a person is hyperactive, quick thinking, and always raring to go. He/she is always up to something and just can't sit still. Their head is full of ideas. Now, if you as a manipulator or people-analyzer do not know this intrinsic fact about the individual's personality, you will most likely misread their body language as nervousness. Tapping their hands and feet, fidgeting with objects, frequently bouncing their legs and more will be viewed as signs of nervousness, when in fact they may be plain restless or wanting to get things done quickly.

If you haven't established a baseline for this person's fundamental personality characteristics, you may end up misreading him or her to conclude that he or she is extremely nervous and not quick-thinking, hyper-energetic and enthusiastic.

You need some background information about a person before determining their thoughts, feelings, and emotions through body language. How does the person generally behave or react in various situations, circumstances, or settings?

How do they generally articulate their thoughts and feelings?

What is their normal voice tone while going through various emotions? Is it different when they are delighted, sad, happy, and excited? How do they reveal their interest or lack of interest in something? All this information will help you read the person in specific settings even more effectively and comprehensively, thus reducing errors when it comes to analyzing people. When a behavior pattern is not consistent with their baseline personality, you can smell something amiss.

Setting or Context

Avoid jumping to a conclusion without taking into consideration the setting or context while reading a person. For example, an individual may be extremely rigid and business-like in the workplace, and casual, gregarious, and leisurely when they meet you outside. The context or setting plays a vital role in determining the behavior of a person. If you read the person outside, you may mistakenly believe them to be someone who is more relaxed and casual about everything, which may not really be the case. It is

Chapter Four: Reading Body Language and Analyzing People

simply the setting that encourages him or her to relax.

The context also plays an important part when it comes to analyzing a person. People may simply cross their arms while sitting because they may be feeling cold and not because they are disinterested or mistrustful of what you are saying. In such a scenario, make the environment more comfortable, or the act of folding their arms and legs will also lead to them switching off from what you are saying on a subconscious level.

Sometimes, people may lean in the opposite direction not because they are trying to escape or are disinterested in the conversation but simply because their seating is uncomfortable. Rubbing their nose may not always be a sign of lying—it can be just cold too. This is why you should look for a bunch of clues (more on it in the next point) to arrive at a near accurate conclusion.

Similarly, look at a variety of non-verbal signals to read the person correctly. Consider everything from a person's body language to their voice to the intonation to understand what they are feeling or thinking. The reading becomes even more power-packed if you add verbal communication or a person's choice of words and phrases to the reading.

The setting is extremely important while reading a person. For example, a person is being interviewed for a position. They may be nervous as people generally are during a job interview. In such a situation, they may not maintain eye contact or move their hand over their face several times (out of nervousness). This doesn't necessarily mean he or she is not speaking the truth or resorting to deception. It simply means they are nervous in the high-pressure setting of a job interview.

Look for a Bunch of Clues

One of the biggest blunders people make while reading or analyzing people is to single out clues rather than study them as a cluster. Avoid looking for isolated, standalone clues and look for a group of clues. For instance, if you read about establishing eye contact as a sign of honesty, trust, and authenticity solely by the fact that an individual is not maintaining consistent eye contact, you may quickly to jump to the conclusion that he or she is a liar.

Chapter Four: Reading Body Language and Analyzing People

On the other side, only by the fact that a person maintains consistent eye contact throughout the conversation, you may falsely deduce that he or she is a confident person who is speaking the truth.

You may ignore all other non-verbal signals such as increased perspiration, twitching toes and hands touching the face frequently to falsely conclude that the person is, in fact, telling the truth simply because he or she is maintaining eye contact. To arrive at an accurate reading about a person's thought patterns, feelings, or emotions; you need to consider a cluster of clues including their expressions, posture, walk, voice, features, and more.

It may be easy to mislead people with a single clue, but it is near impossible to fake all the signals together. The process happens at a very subconscious level, and it is not possible to focus on faking every aspect of our non-verbal behavior to throw others off guard. Therefore, when you are reading a person with the intention of manipulating them to get what you want them to do, look for a cluster of clues that help you read them more reliably.

Manipulation

Cultural Context

Some expressions and gestures such as smiling, eye contact and several other non-verbal signals are universal. They mean the same and are understood across multiple cultures as having similar connotations. However, there are certain gestures, movements, and expressions that have different interpretations across cultures. You this may lead to you misreading another person's thought patterns or emotions based on the non-verbal signals within your culture. Have a clear cultural baseline for reading people's behavior, so you don't end up analyzing it through the filter of your culture.

For example, people in the Italian culture are believed to be loud, gregarious and vivacious in the manner through which they express themselves. Their gestures are animated and enthusiastic. They also speak in an excited, high pitched tone, marked by exuberant screaming and shouting. This is the manner through which they communicate their excitement, delight, and affection.

Someone who comes from Great Britain or another more restrained culture where

Chapter Four: Reading Body Language and Analyzing People

excitement or enthusiasm is more underplayed may not be able to interpret these non-verbal signs accurately. When you view a person's verbal and non-verbal communication patterns in a cultural frame, it becomes simpler to read them correctly.

Even similar gestures can have different interpretations across cultures. For example, a thumbs-up gesture can represent validation or best wishes in western countries. However, the same thumbs-up sign is not considered a culturally appropriate gesture in some Middle Eastern regions. It is seen as rude and inappropriate.

Chapter Five:
Secret Social and Subconscious Manipulation Strategies

While manipulators are generally consciously and purposefully aggressive while fulfilling their agenda, the most dangerous form of manipulation is subconscious manipulation. It occurs at a deeper level and preys on the victim's psychological feelings unlike conscious manipulation where the person dominates, screams, and lies to get what they want.

Why does subconscious manipulation go undetected?

The techniques are subtle and not explicit.

Victims of subconscious manipulation may have a gut reaction or even unpleasant feeling about the manipulator. However, since it isn't explicit or they aren't able to consciously recognize it, they can't logically explain the dynamics of what they are experiencing.

The tactics are often disguised in a more positive garb.

A master subconscious manipulator or persuader may alter their behavior into demonstrating that they are caring, kind, concerned, or crusading to hide their negative agenda. For instance, if the victim reacts negatively to your insults or subtle subconscious attacks, you label them hypersensitive or overly emotional, which they fight challenging to defend.

It is precisely for this reason that manipulation victims are led to feel weak, insecure and uncertain about their beliefs. This leaves them weak and open, which only allows you, as a manipulator, to penetrate deeper into their subconscious.

Exploiting weaknesses

Manipulators will continuously exploit a person's weaknesses and insecurities to exploit them to fulfill their agenda. They will rationalize it as something that the victim deserves. The victims

Chapter Five: Secret Social and Subconscious Manipulation Strategies

generally become blind to their weaknesses or insecurities and completely deny that someone is taking advantage of them. People generally lack the self-knowledge to detect or face their own subconscious vulnerabilities, which you as a manipulator can cash in on. For instance, a buyer who has fallen for a sales tactic will tend to rationalize or justify their purchase over-analyzing their own deep-seated subconscious vulnerability.

Here's looking at some secret and covert manipulation techniques that are widely used by master manipulators to persuade people into doing what they (the manipulators wants).

Create Problems and Offer Solutions

This is a favorite social and subconscious manipulation technique used by master manipulators across the world. As a manipulator, you create an imaginary problem or issue for creating or stimulating a particular reaction from the victim or public at large. The manipulator then sneakily introduces a solution to the problem he or she himself or herself has created.

Manipulation

For instance, first political outfits may allow city violence or fringe terrorist groups to thrive by cleverly overlooking their activities. This will be quickly followed by bringing about an awareness of how people's security is the administration or political outfit's primary concern. They will focus on how they will go all out for strengthening security measures for ensuring public safety.

Manipulators cleverly create a problem and then present a solution for their problems without letting anyone realize that they are responsible for constructing the problems in the first place to come across as heroes for solving people's problems. You become a solution provider this way, which makes it easier for you to get people to act in a certain manner.

The Bitter Pill or Painful Reality

Consider this example carefully to understand how it works as a subconscious level. Your manager urges everyone within the organization to do overtime or pitch in addition work hours. You'll not have to stay up late post work and sometimes even come to the office during weekends. Bitter? Yes of course!

Chapter Five: Secret Social and Subconscious Manipulation Strategies

However, this will be quickly followed up by leading the workforce to believe that there is a high chance of people being laid off within the organization. If people want to keep their jobs, they will have to step up and cover that extra mile for surviving. As a manipulator, your boss may drown you with facts and statistics about how companies who haven't worked on large projects were unable to sustain their operation and other costs and ultimately closed down.

Manipulators often present a situation where they want to get people to do what they want as a bitter pill that has to be taken for the overall good. In the above example, the managers will persuade you about how your sacrifices can have a huge impact in safeguarding the company's future. This again works on a very subconscious level to project something that causes discomfort as a necessary evil. The manipulator will go on about how they don't really want to do something, but there is just no other way out.

Be a Skilled Debater and Public Speaker

Skilled debaters and public speakers find it easy to influence people on a subconscious level through their words. They can prey on people's subconscious feelings and influence them into taking the required action.

Sign up for a public speaking class if you want to be a master manipulator or develop people-convincing skills. You will develop the ability to communicate your ideas in a compelling, assertive, authoritative, arresting, and impressive manner.

Have you ever noticed how some of history's best speakers were able to hypnotize people through their speeches accompanied by the right non-verbal signals? People utilize everything from the tone of their voice to their gestures to the right actions and words to influence people in a specific direction of thought.

Observe how influencers and powerful leaders use their voice and tone to leave behind the right impression.

Conclusion

Thank you again for buying this book!

I hope this book was able to help you understand the basic and advanced manipulation techniques and how they can be used in your daily life to get exactly what you want.

The next step is to simply use all the tried and tested strategies, tips, and techniques mentioned in this valuable resource to control people's minds and influence them into doing what you want them to without them even realizing it.

The book is packed with practical tips, real-life examples and proven strategies to help you get a good grip of the art of manipulation, and how to use it resourcefully to get people to feel, think, and behave in a manner you want them to.

Finally, if you enjoyed this book, then I'd like to ask you for a favor, would you be kind enough to leave a review for this book on Amazon? It'd be greatly appreciated!

Manipulation

Thank you and good luck!

www.ingramcontent.com/pod-product-compliance
Lightning Source LLC
Chambersburg PA
CBHW020912080526
44589CB00011B/565